The Banting Diet: Letter on Corpulence

ALSO BY WILL MEADOWS

The Final Countdown Diet

The Banting Diet: Letter on Corpulence

By

William Banting

With a Foreword & Commentary

By

Will Meadows

Published by FCD Publishing

First Published 2015

ISBN: 1507585810

ISBN-13: 978-1507585818

To J, W, B & C – simply for being there.

CONTENTS

1   Introduction   1

2   Foreword & Commentary   3

3   Letter on Corpulence   15

4   Preface to the Third Edition   17

5   Corpulence   21

6   Concluding Addenda   44

7   Appendix   54

8   Preface to the Fourth Edition   59

9   About The Authors   81

DISCLAIMER

The material in this book is intended solely for informational purposes only. It consists of a reproduction of a historical document and associated commentary. It does not constitute diet advice. You should always consult a doctor if you wish to begin a diet plan. The author and publisher expressly disclaim any responsibility for any adverse effects that may result from the use or misuse of the information and advice contained within this book.

WILLIAM BANTING

INTRODUCTION

Long before the Atkins Diet and the steady stream of copycat low carbohydrate diets that followed came a diet book that was written – not by Doctors or nutritionists – but by a humble Victorian undertaker. This diet would pave the way for many of the diets that followed over the next 150 years. Importantly it would serve to imprint the 'low carb' mindset into the consciousness of the dieting public. That Victorian undertaker was William Banting and the account of his weight loss, detailed in *Letter on Corpulence*, is arguably the most important diet book ever written.

I have been involved in the diet and nutrition industries for many years and it is impossible to escape the impact that Banting's work has had on people's lives. The foundations he laid for a low carb existence have informed many of the diets we find popular today. My own diet book, *The Final Countdown Diet* - whilst not a low carb diet book - could not have been written without the contribution that Banting made to the science of weight loss. Put simply, Banting paved the way for the diet phenomenon that we see today. It is therefore with great pleasure that I provide the foreword, commentary and accompanying notes to *The Third Edition* of William Banting's *Letter on Corpulence*.

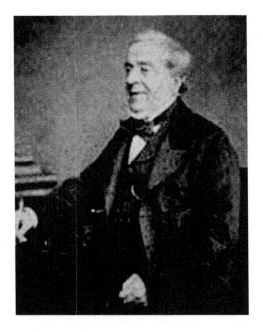

William Banting (1796-1878)

FOREWORD & COMMENTARY

In the late nineteenth century a new verb entered the English language. The verb 'to bant' meant that a person was on a diet. When that person began to lose weight, they were said to be 'banting'. Although use of the words 'bant' and 'banting' declined in the twentieth century, these words can still be found in some dictionaries to the present day. The source of these new words was an elderly Victorian undertaker named William Banting. In 1885 the Dictionary of National Biography described him as follows - 'somewhat short of stature' and 'suffering great personal inconvenience from his increasing fatness'. At a height of only 5 ft 5 inches tall and a weight of 202 lbs, Banting was considered to be very fat by the standards of Victorian Britain. Indeed, even by today's standards Banting would be medically classified as obese.

Banting did not come from a family with a propensity to obesity. In fact in Victorian times obesity was relatively rare. Remarkably the calorific intake of the average Victorian citizen was far higher than that of today – some 50%-100% higher[1]. Certain factors however were at play to prevent the average Victorian worker from becoming obese. One factor was the level of activity undertaken - Victorian workers were active for 55 to 70 hours a week. Not only that, their diet was of a surprisingly high quality and contained a variety of fresh, unprocessed and nutritious foods. A person of Banting's size would therefore be unusual and it would appear from his writings that this made him the subject of much ridicule.

It would seem that part of Banting's weight problem echoes the problems we face in today's society. He was relatively wealthy and had a largely sedentary lifestyle. He also lived at a time when processed foods, and sugars, were entering the diets of those who could afford them. Banting had made attempts to lose weight in the past and had sought advice from various doctors. However the advice he received led to Banting entering what he describes as a 'low impoverished state'. This condition caused 'many obnoxious boils to appear' as well as 'carbuncles'. Although undiagnosed at the time, it's likely that the result of Banting's previous trip to the

---

[1] Clayton P & Rowbotham J, (2009) "How the Mid-Victorians Worked, Ate and Died", *International Journal of Environmental Research and Public Health*. Mar 2009; 6(3): 1235–1253

Doctors was a course of treatment that had led to malnutrition – carbuncles being firmly associated with such an ailment.

On 26th August 1862, at the age of sixty-five, William Banting woke from his sleep in his London home. With some difficulty he attended to his morning ablutions and dressed himself for the day ahead. Once dressed, he began the journey downstairs – this would take some time. Due to his size and various ailments, Banting had to descend the stairs backwards and very slowly. This was the only method he had found to reduce the strain on his knee and ankle joints. He arrived at the bottom of the stairs puffing and blowing.

After a breakfast of buttered toast washed down with a pint of milky and sugary tea, Banting made his way to his front door and with great difficulty tied his shoes – being unable to stoop down low enough. Once his shoes were tied, he opened the door and ventured outside. He had a Doctor's appointment that day - and he couldn't be late.

Banting was on his way to meet Dr William Harvey, an eminent ear, nose and throat specialist. The aim of the appointment was to find a remedy for Banting's failing sight and increasing deafness. The outcome of the meeting was something altogether more momentous. Dr

Harvey realised that Banting's overall health condition may well be the result of his obesity. Dr Harvey immediately put Banting on a diet, the aim of the diet was to reduce Banting's consumption of 'saccharine' (sugars) and starch.

Over the next year by following Dr. Harvey's advice, Banting lost an average of just under 1lb per week. At the end of that first year, Banting had lost 46 lbs in weight. Not only that, his sight and hearing had improved and he was finally able to tackle the stairs at home with ease. Banting was not the first patient that Dr. Harvey had tried this remedy on. An earlier patient - also obese and suffering from deafness - had been given the same eating regime. That patient also experienced remarkable weight loss combined with the elimination of his hearing problems.

Perhaps this remarkable diet would have been lost to history had Banting not been an industrious and philanthropic soul. Banting had a great desire to see others cured from the 'disease' of obesity. It is perhaps fair to say that Banting was well known in Victorian society. Although he was an undertaker – he wasn't just *any* undertaker – he was the undertaker to Royalty! Banting had personally conducted the funerals of Prince Albert and the Duke of Wellington and his family would go on to bury Queen Victoria. With unquestionable connections in society and an evident flair for marketing, Banting set about publishing the principles of Dr Harvey's diet in his

'Letter on Corpulence'. It became an overnight sensation.

Although *Letter on Corpulence* certainly wasn't the first diet book in the world - many 'reducing' diets had been published before - it was the first diet book that worked. What's more, it didn't rely unnecessarily on extreme measures or mysterious potions[2]. In line with his philanthropic aims, the first editions of the book were given away for free. Later editions were sold so that his costs could be covered. Any profit was donated to charitable causes.

Interestingly, Banting's efforts to provide a 'solution' to the obesity problem were met with stern resistance from the medical profession. Banting firmly believed that his various medical ailments were clearly linked to obesity however he was constantly advised by medical practitioners that obesity (or 'corpulence') was in fact 'incurable'. One able physician advised Banting that he himself 'had gained 1 lb in weight every year since he attained manhood' with the advice to do a bit more

---

[2] Although Banting's food regime is clearly documented, there is less information about the accompanying 'draught' or alkaline drink prescribed by Dr. Harvey. Banting states that this concoction's purpose was to remove all the 'dregs left in the stomach after digestion' although he points out that it was not a laxative.

exercise and take more vapour-baths and shampooing[3]. Whilst the advice to bath and shampoo might be laughable today, exercise is still frequently prescribed for those wishing to lose weight. However, as explained in my own book *The Final Countdown Diet*, exercise is a totally inefficient method of losing weight. Not least for what Banting describes as the after-effect of working up a 'prodigious appetite'. Luckily, in Dr. Harvey, Banting found a medical practitioner able to offer sound advice. But how does that advice stand up to the test of time?

A study conducted in 1993 for the journal *Obesity Research*[4] concluded that Banting's personal daily diet was a low-carbohydrate, high protein, high-fat diet containing in the region of 1700 calories. Within the United Kingdom the current recommended calorific intake to maintain weight is 2500 Kcal a day. On this basis Banting would be in a calorific deficit of 800 calories a day. As discussed in my own diet publication, *The Final Countdown Diet*, mere calorific deficit is only part of the weight loss story. Importantly for the success of Banting's diet, not only was

[3] The observation that weight increases with age still rings true today. Research conducted in America by the National Institutes of Health's National Heart, Lung and Blood Institute has shown that people aged 18-49 gain an average of 1-2 lbs each year with larger gains occurring in 20-29 year olds. (NIH, N.H.L and Blood Institute, November 2010, *Trials use technology to help young adults achieve healthy weights*).

[4] Bray, G (1993) "Commentary on Banting Letters", *Obesity Research* Vol 1 (2) Mar 93

he reducing his calories, he was also restricting 'saccharine' and starches - known today as simple and complex carbohydrates.

As a result of restricting his intake of carbohydrates, Banting was lessening the chance of any excess carbohydrates being stored as fat by the body. It was this carbohydrate restriction combined with an overall calorific deficit that led to the remarkable weight loss experienced by Banting. Interestingly, Banting concluded from his own personal experiments that 'saccharine matter is the great moving cause of fatty corpulence'. Identifying sugar as the 'bad guy' was clearly a thought process that was ahead of its time. Only very recently has medical opinion begun to shift towards sugar being the main cause of obesity rather than fat. Put simply, fat doesn't make you fat – sugar does.

Restricting all things 'saccharine' also led to Dr. Harvey advising against the consumption of milk. Dr. Harvey was quite correct in this advice as milk contains lactose: a simple sugar. This advice resulted in Banting drinking his daily ration of tea without milk. What he and Dr Harvey could never have realized is that this method of drinking tea would actually help in Banting's weight loss. Tea contains certain compounds called theaflavins and thearubigins which have been shown to prevent obesity in various scientific studies[5]. However when you add milk to tea, these fat-fighting compounds are effectively neutralized[6]. When Banting started to drink his tea without milk he was unwittingly increasing the ability of his body to fight fat.

However it's not all good news. There are some dangers in following a low carbohydrate, high protein, high fat diet that would not have been known in Banting's time. Such diets have been linked with kidney problems, ketosis and high cholesterol - amongst other ailments. Banting however seemed to thrive on such a diet. Why might this be? It is perhaps important to note that, by the time of the Third Edition of *Letter on Corpulence*, Banting was readily acknowledging that he was no longer strictly maintaining his diet regime. From time he would allow himself to indulge in whatever treats he fancied and frequently enjoyed all of the previously 'banned' items – with the exception of beer. That said, Banting remained mindful of the importance of keeping a check on such activity and would not allow any such indulgences to get out of control. In fact, Banting took such deviations as a source

---

[5] Satoshi U, Yoshimasa T & Akiko Saka et al (2010) "Prevention of diet-induced obesity by dietary black tea polyphenols extract in vitro and in vivo" *Nutrition.* Vol 27, Issue 3: 287-292

[6] Research conducted by Devajit Borthakur, a scientist at the Tea Research Association in Assam, India in 2011

of satisfaction, confident that he held 'the power of maintaining the happy medium (i.e. his weight)' in his own hands.

In line with some of the dangers of the Banting Diet, some of Dr. Harvey's advice can also be queried – such as avoiding salmon and oily fish. These days we are well aware of the benefits to be gained from consuming the Omega-3 fatty acids contained within such fish. These benefits include the prevention of cardiovascular disease and a reduction in the risk of contracting rheumatoid arthritis. We can only speculate on the reasons behind such dietary advice although it's clear that Dr. Harvey believed such fish had a 'fattening character' similar to that he believed was contained in Pork. Such transgressions however can be easily forgiven with the benefit of 150 years of hindsight!

Banting identified a weight loss factor within his diet that is also common with the low carb diets of today. He noted that the greatest 'diminution in weight and bulk occurs within the first forty-eight hours' with more gradual weight loss thereafter. Banting believed that this was mother nature doing her duty and getting rid of 'immediate pressure' which then allowed her to 'move more freely in her own beautiful way'. With the benefit of a 21st Century viewpoint we can determine that this initial weight loss is purely the result of the loss of body water and not the work of nature relieving her pressure. This is a natural reaction of our bodies expending our glycogen reserves and dispensing with the water used in glycogen storage. Certain 'quick fix' diet companies still use this 'false' weight loss today to erroneously claim rapid results.

Banting's emphasis on gradual weight loss exactly matches my own views that, for weight loss to be sustainable, it needs to take place over the medium to long-term. In our present-day society we are accustomed to instant gratification. If we want to lose weight we want to see remarkable results in a short timeframe. However such 'quick fix' or 'fad' diets invariably end up with people being heavier than when they started. In fact studies have shown that most people who diet will regain all the weight they lost[7]. The fact that Banting managed to consistently lose around a 1 lb of weight every week for a year – and that he managed to keep that weight off - calls into question our current obsession with instantaneous diet results. It would seem, again, that Banting was 150 years ahead of the game when he correctly identified that 'it cannot but be dangerous…to reduce a disease of this nature suddenly'.

I hope you enjoy this edition of Banting's seminal *Letter on Corpulence* along with the accompanying notes I have provided. I believe this document provides a fascinating insight into Victorian attitudes towards what

---

[7] Sumithran, P & Proietto, J (2013) "The defence of body weight: a physiological basis for weight regain after weight loss": *Clinical Science (2013) 124*

Banting termed the 'disease' of corpulence. Although our language may have changed somewhat since Victorian times and 'corpulence' is no longer part of the vernacular, its modern-day equivalent – obesity – remains a problem to which there seem to be few easy answers.

Will Meadows
West Yorkshire
2015

WILLIAM BANTING

LETTER

ON CORPULENCE,

Addressed to the Public

By WILLIAM BANTING.

THIRD EDITION.

LONDON:

PUBLISHED BY HARRISON, 59, PALL MALL,

Bookseller to the Queen and H.R.H. the Prince of Wales.

1864.

WILLIAM BANTING

PREFACE TO THE THIRD EDITION

The second edition of this pamphlet (consisting of 1,500 copies) being exhausted, and the result being very gratifying to my mind, in the large amount of satisfaction and benefit which I am able to report from evidence of others (*beyond my most sanguine expectations*), considering the hitherto limited circulation, I have felt impelled to pubhsh, advertise, and sell this third edition, at cost price, which I am informed must be sixpence a copy. If this small charge, however, should yield any profit, I shall devote it to the Printers' Pension Society, or some other benevolent institution; but I have no such expectation, or would very gladly reduce the charge at starting.

The first and second editions were no very serious expense to me, scarcely three pence a copy, but the circulation of them, and the correspondence involved, have cost me far more; yet, I saw no way of securing my motives from misconception except by gratuitously presenting the pamphlet to the public.

The truthful tale has, however, made its way into a large circle of sufferers with marvellous effect; and I can now believe the public will rather prefer to purchase the third edition at a reasonable charge than be under obligation to me for a gratuitous supply. I therefore humbly trust, and fully believe, that by this means the useful knowledge will be distributed twenty-fold to the benefit of suffering humanity, which, indeed, is my sole object.

Kensington,
  December, 1863.

This letter is respectfully dedicated to the Public simply and entirely from an earnest desire to confer a benefit on my fellow creatures.

W. B.

WILLIAM BANTING

CORPULENCE

Of all the parasites that affect humanity I do not know of, nor can I imagine, any more distressing than that of Obesity, and, having just emerged from a very long probation in this affliction, I am desirous of circulating my humble knowledge and experience for the benefit of my fellow man, with an earnest hope it may lead to the same comfort and happiness I now feel under the extraordinary change, which might almost be termed miraculous had it not been accomplished by the most simple common-sense means.

Obesity seems to me very little understood or properly appreciated by the faculty and the public generally, or the former would long ere this have hit upon the cause for so lamentable a disease, and applied effective remedies, whilst the latter would have spared their injudicious indulgence in remarks and sneers, frequently painful in society, and which, even on the strongest mind, have an unhappy tendency; but I sincerely trust this humble effort at exposition may lead to a more perfect ventilation of the subject and a better feeling for the afflicted.

It would afford me infinite pleasure and satisfaction to name the author of my redemption from the calamity, as he is the only one that I have been able to find (and my search has not been sparing) who seems thoroughly up in the question but such publicity might be construed improperly, and I have, therefore, only to offer my personal experience as the stepping-stone to public investigation, and to proceed with my narrative of facts, earnestly hoping the reader will patiently peruse and thoughtfully consider it, with forbearance for any fault of style or diction, and for any seeming presumption in publishing it.

I have felt some difficulty in deciding on the proper and best course of action. At one time I thought the Editor of the Lancet would kindly publish a letter from me on the subject, but further reflection led me to doubt whether an insignificant individual would be noticed without some special introduction. In the April number of the *Cornhill Magazine* I read with much interest an article on the subject - defining tolerably well the effects, but ofiering no tangible remedy, or even positive solution of the problem - "What is the Cause of Obesity?" I was pleased with the article as a whole, but objected to some portions, and had prepared a letter to the Editor of that Magazine ofiering my experience on the subject, but again it struck me that an unknown individual like myself would have but little prospect of notice; so I finally resolved to publish and circulate this Pamphlet, with no other reason, motive, or expectation than an earnest desire to help those who happen to be afflicted as I was, for that corpulence is remediable I am well convinced, and shall be delighted if I can induce others to think so. The object I have in view impels me to enter into minute particulars as well as general observations, and to revert to bygone years, in order to show that I have spared no pains nor expense to accomplish the great end of stopping and curing obesity.

I am now nearly 66 years of age, about 5 feet 5 inches in stature, and, in August last (1862), weighed 202 lbs., which I think it right to name, because the article in the *Cornhill Magazine* presumes that a certain stature and age should bear ordinarily a certain weight, and I am quite of that opinion. I now weigh 167 lbs., showing a diminution of something like 1 lb. per week since August, and having now very nearly attained the happy medium, I have perfect confidence that a few more weeks will fully accomplish the object for which I have laboured for the last thirty years, in vain, until it pleased Almighty Providence to direct me into the right and proper channel - the "tramway," so to speak - of happy, comfortable existence.

Few men have led a more active life - bodily or mentally - from a constitutional anxiety for regularity, precision, and order, during fifty years' business career, from which I have now retired, so that my corpulence and subsequent obesity was not through neglect of necessary bodily activity, nor from excessive eating, drinking, or self-indulgence of any kind, except that I partook of the simple aliments of bread, milk, butter, beer, sugar, and potatoes more freely than my aged nature required, and hence, as I believe, the generation of the parasite, detrimental to comfort if not really to health.

I will not presume to descant on the bodily structural tissues, so fully canvassed in the *Cornhill Magazine*, nor how they are supported and renovated, having no mind or power to enter into those questions, which properly belong to the wise heads of the faculty. None of my family on the side of either parent had any tendency to corpulence, and from my earliest years I had an inexpressible dread of such a calamity, so, when I was between thirty and forty years of age, finding a tendency to it creeping upon me, I consulted an eminent surgeon, now long deceased, - a kind personal friend, - who recommended increased bodily exertion before my ordinary daily labours began, and thought rowing an excellent plan. I had the command of a good, heavy, safe boat, lived near the river, and adopted it for a couple of hours in the early morning. It is true I gained muscular vigour, but with it a prodigious appetite, which I was compelled to indulge, and consequently increased in weight, until my kind old friend advised me to forsake the exercise.

He soon afterwards died, and, as the tendency to corpulence remained, I consulted other high orthodox authorities (*never any inferior adviser*), but all in vain. I have tried sea air and bathing in various localities, with much walking exercise; taken gallons of physic and liquor potassae, advisedly and abundantly; riding on horseback; the waters and climate of Leamington many times, as well as those of Cheltenham and Harrogate frequently; have lived upon sixpence a-day, so to speak, and earned it, if bodily labour may be so construed ; and have spared no trouble nor expense in consultations with the best authorities in the land, giving each and all a fair time for experiment, without any permanent remedy, as the evil still gradually increased.

I am under obligations to most of those advisers for the pains and interest they took in my case; but only to one for an effectual remedy.

When a corpulent man eats, drinks, and sleeps well, has no pain to complain of, and no particular organic disease, the judgment of able men seems paralyzed - for I have been generally informed that corpulence is one of the natural results of increasing years; indeed, one of the ablest authorities as a physician in the land told me he had gained

1 lb. in weight every year since he attained manhood, and was not surprised at my condition, but advised more bodily exercise - vapour-baths and shampooing, in addition to the medicine given. Yet the evil still increased, and, like the parasite of barnacles on a ship, if it did not destroy the structure, it obstructed its fair, comfortable progress in the path of life.

I have been in dock, perhaps twenty times in as many years, for the reduction of this disease, and with little good effect - none lasting. Any one so afflicted is often subject to public remark, and though in conscience he may care little about it, I am confident no man labouring under obesity can be quite insensible to the sneers and remarks of the cruel and injudicious in public assemblies, public vehicles, or the ordinary street traffic; nor to the annoyance of finding no adequate space in a public assembly if he should seek amusement or need refreshment, and therefore he naturally keeps away as much as possible from places where he is likely to be made the object of the taunts and remarks of others. I am as regardless of public remark as most men, but I have felt these difficulties and therefore avoided such circumscribed accommodation and notice, and by that means have been deprived of many advantages to health and comfort.

Although no very great size or weight, still I could not stoop to tie my shoe, so to speak, nor attend to the little offices humanity requires without considerable pain and difficulty, which only the corpulent can understand; I have been compelled to go down stairs slowly backwards, to save the jarr of increased weight upon the ancle and knee joints, and been obliged to puff and blow with every slight exertion, particularly that of going up stairs. I have spared no pains to remedy this by low living (*moderation and light food* was generally prescribed, but I had no direct bill of fare to know what was really intended), and that, consequently, brought the system into a low impoverished state, without decreasing corpulence, caused many obnoxious boils to appear, and two rather formidable carbuncles, for which I was ably operated upon *and fed into increased obesity.*

At this juncture (about three years back) Turkish baths became the fashion, and I was advised to adopt them as a remedy. With the first few I found immense benefit in power and elasticity for walking exercise; so, believing I had found the "philosopher's stone," pursued them three times a-week till I had taken fifty, then less frequently (as I began to fancy, with some reason, that so many weakened my constitution) till I had taken ninety, but never succeeded in losing more than 6 lbs. weight during the whole course, and I gave up the plan as worthless; though I have full belief in their cleansing properties, and their value in colds, rheumatism, and many other ailments.

I then fancied increasing obesity materially

affected a slight umbilical rapture, if it did not cause it, and that another bodily ailment to which I had been subject was also augmented. This led me to other medical advisers, to whom I am also indebted for much kind consideration, though, unfortunately, they failed in relieving me. At last finding my sight failing and my hearing greatly impaired, I consulted in August last an eminent aural surgeon, who made light of the case, looked into my ears, sponged them internally, and blistered the outside, without the slightest benefit, neither inquiring into any of my bodily ailments, which he probably thought unnecessary, nor affording me even time to name them.

I was not at all satisfied, but on the contrary was in a worse plight than when I went to him; however he soon after left town for his annual holiday, which proved the greatest possible blessing to me, because it compelled me to seek other assistance, and, happily, I found the right man, who unhesitatingly said he believed my ailments were caused principally by corpulence, and prescribed a certain diet, - no medicine, beyond a morning cordial as a corrective - with immense effect and advantage both to my hearing and the decrease of my corpulency.

For the sake of argument and illustration I will presume that certain articles of ordinary diet, however beneficial in youth, are prejudicial in advanced life, like beans to a horse, whose common ordinary food is hay and corn. It may be useful food occasionally, under peculiar circumstances, but detrimental as a constancy. I will, therefore, adopt the analogy, and call such food human beans. The items from which I was advised to abstain as much as possible were:- Bread, butter, milk, sugar, beer, and potatoes, which had been the main (and, I thought, innocent) elements of my existence, or at all events they had for many years been adopted freely.

These, said my excellent adviser, contain starch and saccharine matter, tending to create fat, and should be avoided altogether. At the first blush it seemed to me that I had little left to live upon, but my kind friend soon showed me there was ample, and I was only too happy to give the plan a fair trial, and, within a very few days, found immense benefit from it. It may better elucidate the dietary plan if I describe generally what I have sanction to take, and that man must be an extraordinary person who would desire a better table:-

For breakfast, I take four or five ounces of beef, mutton, kidneys, broiled fish, bacon, or cold meat of any kind except pork; a large cup of tea (without milk or sugar), a little biscuit, or one ounce of dry toast.

For dinner, Five or six ounces of any fish except salmon, any meat except pork, any vegetable except potato, one ounce of dry toast, fruit out of a pudding, any kind of poultry or game, and two or three glasses of good claret, sherry, or Madeira - Champagne, Port and Beer are forbidden.

For tea, Two or three ounces of fruit, a rusk or two, and a cup of tea without milk or sugar.

For supper, Three or four ounces of meat or fish, similar to dinner, with a glass or two of claret.

For nightcap, if required, A tumbler of grog
- (gin, whisky, or brandy, without sugar)
- or a glass or two of claret or sherry.

This plan leads to an excellent night's rest, with from six to eight hours' sound sleep. The dry toast or rusk may have a table spoonful of spirit to soften it, which will prove acceptable. Perhaps I did not wholly escape starchy or saccharine matter, but scrupulously avoided those beans, such as milk, sugar, beer, butter, &c., which were known to contain them.

On rising in the morning I take a table spoonful of a special corrective cordial, which may be called the Balm of life, in a wine-glass of water, a most grateful draught, as it seems to carry away all the dregs left in the stomach after digestion, but is not aperient; then I take about 5 or 6 ounces solid and 8 of liquid for breakfast ; 8 ounces of solid and 8 of liquid for dinner ; 3 ounces of solid and 8 of liquid for tea; 4 ounces of solid and 6 of liquid for supper, and the grog afterwards, if I please. I am not, however, strictly limited to any quantity at either meal, so that the nature of the food is rigidly adhered to.

Experience has taught me to believe that these human beans are the most insidious enemies man, with a tendency to corpulence in advanced life, can possess, though eminently friendly to youth. He may very prudently mount guard against such an enemy if he is not a fool to himself, and I fervently hope this truthful unvarnished tale may lead him to make a trial of my plan, which I sincerely recommend to public notice, - not with any ambitious motive, but in sincere good faith to help my fellow-creatures to obtain the marvellous blessings I have found within the short period of a few months.

I do not recommend every corpulent man to rush headlong into such a change of diet, (*certainly not*), but to act advisedly and after full consultation with a physician.

My former dietary table was bread and milk for breakfast, or a pint of tea with plenty of milk and sugar,and buttered toast; meat, beer, much bread (of which I was always very fond) and pastry for dinner, the meal of tea similar to that of breakfast, and generally a fruit tart or bread and milk for supper. I had little comfort and far less sound sleep.

It certainly appears to me that my present dietary table is far superior to the former — more luxurious and liberal, independent of its blessed effect - but when it is proved to be more healthful, comparisons are simply ridiculous, and I can hardly imagine any man, even in sound health, would choose the former, even if it were not an enemy; but, when it is shown to be, as in my case, inimical both to health and comfort, I can hardly conceive there is any man who would not willingly avoid it. I can conscientiously assert I never lived so well as under the new plan of dietary, which I should have formerly thought a dangerous extravagant trespass upon health; I am very much better, bodily and mentally, and pleased to believe that I hold the reins of health and comfort in my own hands, and, though at sixty-five years of age, I cannot expect to remain free from some coming natural infirmity that all flesh is heir to, I cannot at the present time complain of one. It is simply miraculous, and I am thankful to Almighty Providence for directing me, through an extraordinary chance, to the care of a man who could work such a change in so short a time.

Oh! that the faculty would look deeper into and make themselves better acquainted with the crying evil of obesity - that dreadful tormenting parasite on health and comfort. Their fellow men might not descend into early premature graves, as I believe many do, from what is termed apoplexy, and certainly would not, during their sojourn on earth, endure so much bodily and consequently mental infirmity.

Corpulence, though giving no actual pain, as it appears to me, must naturally press with undue violence upon the bodily viscera, driving one part upon another, and stopping the free action of all. I am sure it did in my particular case, and the result of my experience is briefly as follows:-

I have not felt so well as now for the last twenty years. Have suffered no inconvenience whatever the probational remedy.

Am reduced many inches in bulk, and 35 lbs. in weight in thirty-eight weeks.

Come down stairs forward naturally, with perfect ease.

Go up stairs and take ordinary exercise freely, without the slightest inconvenience.

Can perform every necessary office for myself

The umbilical rupture is greatly ameliorated, and gives me no anxiety.

My sight is restored — my hearing improved.

My other bodily ailments are ameliorated; indeed,

almost past into matter of history.

I have placed a thank-offering of £50 in the hands of my kind medical adviser for distribution amongst his favourite hospitals, after gladly paying his usual fees, and still remain under overwhelming obligations for his care and attention, which I can never hope to repay. Most thankful to Almighty Providence for mercies received, and determined to press the case into public notice as a token of gratitude.

I have the pleasine to afford, in conclusion, a satisfactory confirmation of my report, in stating that a corpulent friend of mine, who, like myself, is possessed of a generally sound constitution, was laboring under frequent palpitations of the heart and sensations of fainting, was, at my instigation, induced to place himself in the hands of my medical adviser, with the same gradual beneficial results. He is at present under the same ordeal, and in eight weeks has profited even more largely than I did in that short period; he has lost the palpitations, and is becoming, so to speak, a new made man - thankful to me for advising, and grateful to the eminent counsellor to whom I referred him - and he looks forward with good hope to a perfect cure.

I am fully persuaded that hundreds, if not thousands, of our fellow men might profit equally by a similar course; but, constitutions not being all alike, a different course of treatment may be advisable for the removal of so tormenting an affliction.

My kind and valued medical adviser is not a doctor for obesity, but stands on the pinnacle of fame in the treatment of another malady, which, as he well knows, is frequently induced by the disease of which I am speaking, and I most sincerely trust most of my corpulent fiiends (and there are thousands of corpulent people whom I dare not so rank) may be led into my tramroad. To any such I am prepared to offer the further key of knowledge by naming the man. It might seem invidious to do so now, but I shall only be too happy, if applied to by letter in good faith, or if any doubt should exist as to the correctness
of this statement.

WILLIAM BANTING, Sen.,
Late of No. 27, St. James's Street, Piccadilly,
Now of No. 4, The Terrace, Kensington.

May, 1863.

WILLIAM BANTING

ADDENDA

Having exhausted the first Edition (1,000 copies) of the foregoing Pamphlet; and a period of one year having elapsed since connnencing the admirable course of diet which has led to such inestimably beneficial results, and, "as I expected, and desired," having quite succeeded in attaining the happy medium of weight and bulk I had so long ineffectually sought, *which appears necessary to health at my age and stature* - I feel impelled by a sense of public duty, to offer the result of my experience in a second Edition. It has been suggested that I should have sold the Pamphlet, devoting any profit to Charity as more agreeable and useful; and I had intended to adopt such a course, but on reflection feared my motives might be mistaken; I, therefore, respectfully present this (like the first Edition) to the Public gratuitously, earnestly hoping the subject may be taken up by medical men and thoroughly ventilated.

It may (and I hope will) be, as satisfactory to the public to hear, as it is for me to state, that the first Edition has been attended with very comforting results to other sufferers from Corpulence, as the remedial system therein described was to me under that terrible disease, which was my main object in publishing my convictions on the subject. It has moreover attained a success, produced flattering compliments, and an amount of attention I could hardly have imagined possible. The pleasure and satisfaction this has afforded me, is ample compensation for the trouble and expense I have incurred, and I most sincerely trust, "as I verily believe," this second Edition will be accompanied by similar satisfactory results from a more extensive circulation. If so, it will inspire me to circulate further Editions, whilst a corpulent person exists, requiring, as I think, this system of diet, or so long as my motives cannot be mistaken, and are thankfully appreciated.

My weight is reduced 46 lbs., and as the gradual reductions which I am able to show may be interesting to many, I have great pleasure in stating them, believing they serve to demonstrate further the merit of the system pursued.

My weight on 26th August, 1862, was 202 lbs.

	lbs.	lbs.
On 7th September, it was	200, having lost	2
27th September, it was	197, having lost	3 more
19th October, it was	193, having lost	4 more
9th November, it was	190, having lost	3 more
3rd December, it was	187, having lost	3 more
24th December, it was	184, having lost	3 more
14th Jan. 1863, it was	182, having lost	2 more
4th February, it was	180, having lost	2 more
25th February, it was	178, having lost	2 more
18th March, it was	176, having lost	2 more
8th April, it was	173, having lost	3 more
29th April, it was	170, having lost	3 more
20th May, it was	167, having lost	3 more
10th June, it was	164, having lost	3 more
1st July, it was	161, having lost	3 more
22nd July, it was	159, having lost	2 more

12th August, it was 157, having lost	2 more
26th August, it was 156, having lost	1 more
12th September it was 156, having lost	0 more
Total loss of weight.. ..	46 lbs.

My girth is reduced round the waist, in tailor phraseology, 12 1/4 inches, which extent was hardly conceivable even by my own friends, or my respected medical adviser, until I put on my former clothing, over what I now wear, which was a thoroughly convincing proof of the remarkable change. These important desiderata have been attained by the most easy and comfortable means, with but little medicine, and almost entirely by a system of diet, that formerly I should have thought dangerously generous. I am told by all who know me that my personal appearance is greatly improved, and that I seem to bear the stamp of good health; this may be a matter of opinion or friendly remark, but I can honestly assert that I feel restored in health, "bodily and mentally," appear to have more muscular power and vigour, eat and drink with a good appetite, and sleep well. All symptoms of acidity, indigestion, and heartburn (with which I was frequently tormented) have vanished. I have left off using boot hooks, and other such aids which were indispensable, but being now able to stoop with ease and freedom, are unnecessary. I have lost the feeling of *occasional faintness*, and what I think a remarkable blessing and comfort is that I have been able safely to leave off knee bandages, which I had worn necessarily for 20 past years, and given up a truss almost entirely; indeed I believe I might wholly discard it with safety, but am advised to wear it at least occasionally for the present.

Since publishing my Pamphlet, I have felt constrained to send a copy of it to my former medical advisers, and to ascertain their opinions on the subject. They did not dispute or question the propriety of the system, but either dared not venture its practice upon a man of my age, or thought it too great a sacrifice of personal comfort to be generally advised or adopted, and I fancy none of them appeared to feel the fact of the misery of corpulence. One eminent physician, as I before stated, assured me that increasing weight was a necessary result of advancing years; another equally eminent to whom I had been directed by a very friendly third, who had most kindly but ineffectually failed in a remedy, added to my weight in a few weeks instead of abating the evil. These facts lead me to believe the question is not sufficiently observed or even regarded.

The great charm and comfort of the system is, that its effects are palpable within a week of trial, which creates a natural stimulus to persevere for a few weeks more, when the fact becomes established beyond question.

I only intreat all persons suffering from corpulence to make a fair trial for just one clear month, as I am well convinced, they will afterwards pursue a course which yields extraordinary benefit, till entirely and effectually relieved, and be it remembered, by the sacrifice merely of simple, for the advantage of more generous and comforting food. The simple dietary evidently adds fuel to fire, whereas the superior and liberal seems to extinguish it.

I am delighted to be able to assert that I have proved the great merit and advantage of the system by its result in several other cases, similar to my own, and have full confidence that within the next twelve months I shall know of many more cases restored from the disease of corpulence, for I have received the kindest possible letters from many afflicted strangers and friends, as well as similar personal observations from others whom I have conversed with, and assurances from most of them that they will kindly inform me the result for my own private satisfaction. Many are practising the diet after consultation with their own medical advisers; some few have gone to mine, and others are practicing upon their own convictions of the advantages detailed in the Pamphlet, though I recommend all to act advisedly, in case their constitutions should differ. I am, however, so perfectly satisfied of the great unerring benefits of this system of diet, that I shall spare no trouble to circulate my humble experience. The amount and character of my correspondence on the subject has been strange and singular, but most satisfactory to my mind and feelings.

I am now in that happy comfortable state that I should not hesitate to indulge in any fancy in regard to diet, but if I did so should watch the consequences, and not continue any course which might add to weight or bulk and consequent discomfort.

Is not the system suggestive to artists and men of sedentary employment who cannot spare time for exercise, consequently become corpulent, and clog the little muscular action with a superabundance of fat, thus easily avoided ?

Pure genuine bread may be the staff of life as it is termed. It is so, particularly in youth, but I feel certain it is more wholesome in advanced life if thoroughly toasted, as I take it. My impression is, that any starchy or saccharine matter tends to the disease of corpulence in advanced life, and whether it be swallowed in that form or generated in the stomach, that all things tending to these elements should be avoided, of course always under sound medical authority.

WILLIAM BANTING.

CONCLUDING ADDENDA

It is very satisfactory to me to be able to state, that I remained at the same standard of bulk and weight for several weeks after the 26th August, when I attained the happy natural medium, since which time I have varied in weight from two to three pounds, more or less. I have seldom taken the morning draught since that time, and have frequently indulged my fancy, *experimentally*, in using milk, sugar, butter, and potatoes - indeed, I may say all the forbidden articles *except beer,* in moderation, with impunity, but always as an exception, not as a rule. This deviation, however, convinces me that I hold the power of maintaining the happy medium in my own hands.

A kind friend has lately furnished me with a tabular statement in regard to weight as proportioned to stature, which, under present circumstances and the new movement, may be interesting and useful to corpulent readers:-

STATURE. WEIGHT.

5 feet 1 should be 8 stone 8 or 120 lbs.

5 feet 2 should be 9 stone 0 or 126 lbs.

5 feet 3 should be 9 stone 7 or 133 lbs.

5 feet 4 should be 9 stone 10 or 136 lbs.

5 feet 5 should be 10 stone 2 or 142 lbs.

5 feet 6 should be 10 stone 5 or 145 lbs.

5 feet 7 should be 10 stone 8 or 148 lbs.

5 feet 8 should be 11 stone 1 or 155 lbs.

5 feet 9 should be 11 stone 8 or 162 lbs.

5 feet 10 should be 12 stone 1 or 169 lbs.

5 feet 11 should be 12 stone 6 or 174 lbs.

6 feet 0 should be 12 stone 10 or 178lbs.

This tabular statement, taken from a mean average of 2,648 healthy men, was formed and arranged for an Insurance Company by the late Dr. John Hutchinson. It answered as a pretty good standard, and insurances were regulated upon it. His calculations were made upon the volume of air passing in and out of the lungs and this was his guide as to how far the various organs of the body were in health, and the lungs in particular. It may be viewed as some sort of probable rule, yet only as an average, - some in health weighing more by many pounds than others. It must not be looked upon as infallible, but only as a sort of general reasonable guide to Nature's great and mighty work[8].

On a general view of the question I think it may be conceded that a frame of low stature was hardly intended to bear very heavy weight. Judging from this tabular statement I ought to be considerably lighter than I am at present. I shall not, however, covet or aim at such a result, nor, on the other hand, feel alarmed if I decrease a little more in weight and bulk.

I am certainly more sensitive to cold since I have lost the superabundant fat, but this is remediable by another garment, far more agreeable and satisfactory. Many of my friends have said, "Oh! you have done well so far, but take care you don't go too far." I fancy such a circumstance, with such a dietary, very unlikely, if not impossible; but feeling that I have now nearly attained the right standard of bulk and weight proportional to my stature and age (between 10 and 11 stone), I should not

---

[8] This table, when compared to 21st Century guidelines, is an accurate calculation of the desired weight for a male of medium frame. The Body Mass Index has all of these weights within the healthy range.

hesitate to partake of a fattening dietary occasionally, to preserve that happy standard, if necessary; indeed, I am allowed to do so by my medical adviser but I shall always observe a careful watch upon myself to discover the effect, and act accordingly, so that, if I choose to spend a day or two with Dives, so to speak, I must not forget to devote the next to Lazarus.

The remedy may be as old as the hills, as I have since been told, but its application is of very recent date; and it astonishes me that such a light should have remained so long unnoticed and hidden, as not to afford a glimmer to my anxious mind in a search for it during the last twenty years, even in directions where it might have been expected to be known. I would rather presume it is a new light, than that it was purposely hidden merely because the disease of obesity was not immediately dangerous to existence, nor thought to be worthy of serious consideration. Little do the faculty imagine the misery and bitterness to life through the parasite of corpulence or obesity.

I can now confidently say that *quantity* of diet may be safely left to the natural appetite; and that it is the *quality* only, which is essential to abate and cure corpulence. I stated the quantities of my own dietary, because it was part of a truthful report, but some correspondents have doubted whether it should be more or less in their own cases, a doubt which would be better solved by their own appetite, or medical adviser. I have heard a graphic remark by a corpulent man, which may not be inappropriately stated here, *that big houses were not formed with scanty materials.* This, however, is a poor excuse for self indulgence in improper food, or for not consulting medical authority.

The approach of corpulence is so gradual that, until it is far advanced, persons rarely become objects of attention. Many may have even congratulated themselves on their comely appearance, and have not sought advice or a remedy for what they did not consider an evil, for an evil I can say most truly it is, when in much excess, to which point it must, in my opinion arrive, unless obviated by proper means.

Many have wished to know (as future readers may) the nature of the morning draught, or where it could be obtained, but believing it would have been highly imprudent on my part to have presumed that what was proper for my constitution was applicable to all indiscriminately, I could only refer them to a medical adviser for any aid beyond the dietary; assuring them, however, it was not a dram but of an alkaline character.

Some, I believe, would willingly submit to even a violent remedy, so that an immediate benefit could be produced; this is not the object of the treatment, as it cannot but be dangerous, in my humble opinion, to reduce a disease of this nature suddenly; they are probably then too prone to despair of success, and consider it as unalterably connected with their constitution. Many under this feeling doubtless return to their former habits, encouraged so to act by the ill-judged advice of friends who, I am persuaded (from the correspondence I have had on this most interestmg subject) become unthinking accomplices in the destruction of those whom they regard and esteem.

The question of four meals a-day, and the night cap, has been abundantly and amusingly criticized. I ought perhaps to have stated as an excuse for such liberality of diet, that I breakfast between eight and nine o'clock, dine between one and two, take my slight tea meal between five and six, sup at nine, and only take the night cap when inclination directs. My object in naming it at all was, that, as a part of a whole system, it should be known, and to show it is not forbidden to those who are advised that they need such a luxury; nor was it injurious in my case. Some have inquired whether smoking was prohibited. It was not.

It has also been remarked that such a dietary as mine was too good and expensive for a poor man, and that I had wholly lost sight of that class; but a very poor corpulent man is not so frequently met with, inasmuch as the poor cannot afford the simple inexpensive means for creating fat; but when the tendency does exist in that class, I have no doubt it can be remedied by abstinence from the forbidden articles, and a moderate indulgence in such cheap stimulants as may be recommended by a medical adviser, whom they have ample chances of consulting gratuitously.

I have a very strong feeling that gout (another terrible parasite upon humanity) might be greatly relieved, if not cured entirely, by this proper natural dietary, and sincerely hope some person so afflicted may be induced to practice the harmless plan for three months (as I certainly would if the case were my own) to prove it; but not without advice.

My impression from the experiments I have tried on myself of late is, that saccharine matter is the great moving cause of fatty corpulence. I know that it produces in my individual case increased weight and a large amount of flatulence, and believe, that not only sugar, but all elements tending to create saccharine matter in the process of digestion, should be avoided. I apprehend it will be found in bread, butter, milk, beer, Port wine, and Champagne; I have not found starchy matter so troublesome as the saccharine, which, I think, largely increases acidity as well as fat, but, with ordinary care and observation, people will soon find what food rests easiest in the stomach, and avoid that which does not, during the probationary trial of the proposed dietary. Vegetables and ripe or stewed fruit I have found ample aperients. Failing this, medical advice should be sought.

The word *"parasite"* has been much commented upon, as inappropriate to any but a living creeping thing (of course I use the word in a figurative sense, as a burden to the flesh), but if fat is not an insidious creeping enemy, I do not know what is. I should have equally applied the word to gout, rheumatism, dropsy, and many other diseases.

Whereas hitherto the appeals to me to know the name of my medical adviser have been very numerous, I may say hundreds, which I have gladly answered, though forming no small item of the expense incurred, and whereas the very extensive circulation expected of the third edition is likely to lead to some thousands of similar applications, I feel bound, in self-defence, to state that the medical gentleman to whom I am so deeply indebted is Mr. Harvey, Soho Square, London, whom I consulted for deafness. In the first and second editions, I thought that to give his name would appear like a puff, which I know he abhors; indeed, I should prefer not to do so now, but cannot, in justice to myself, incur further probable expense (which I fancy inevitable) besides the personal trouble, for which I cannot afford time, and, therefore, feel no hesitation to refer to him as my guarantee for the truth of the pamphlet.

One material point I should be glad to impress on my corpulent readers - it is, to get accurately weighed at starting upon the fresh system, and continue to do so weekly or monthly, for the change will be so truly palpable by this course of examination, that it will arm them with perfect confidence in the merit and ultimate success of the plan. I deeply regret not having secured a photographic portrait of my original figure in 1862, to place in juxta position with one of my present form. It might have amused some, but certainly would have been very convincing to others, and astonishing to all that such an effect should have been so readily and speedily produced by the simple natural cause of exchanging a meagre for a generous dietary under proper advice.

I shall ever esteem it a great favour if persons relieved and cured, as I have been, will kindly let me know of it; the information will be truly gratifying to my mind. That the system is a great success, I have not a shadow of doubt from the numerous reports sent with thanks by strangers as well as friends from all parts of the kingdom; and I am truly thankful to have been the humble instrument of disseminating the blessing and experience I have attained through able counsel and natural causes by proper perseverance.

I have now finished my task, and trust my humble efforts may prove to be good seed well sown, that will fructify and produce a large harvest of benefit to my fellow creatures. I also hope the faculty generally may be led more extensively to ventilate this question of corpulence or obesity, so that, instead of one, two, or three able practitioners, there may be as many hundreds distributed in the various parts of the United Kingdom. In such case, I am persuaded, that those diseases, like Reverence and Golden Pippins, will be very rare.

APPENDIX

Since publishing the third edition of my Pamphlet, I have earnestly pressed my medical adviser to explain the reasons for so remarkable a result as I and others have experienced from the dietary system he prescribed, and I hope he may find time to do so shortly, as I believe it would be highly interesting to the Faculty and the public generally. He has promised this at his leisure.

Numerous applications having been made to me on points to which I had not alluded, in which my correspondents felt some doubt and interest, I take this opportunity of making some few corrections in my published dietary:-

I ought, "it seems," to have excepted veal, owing to its indigestible quality, as well as pork for its fattening character; also herrings and eels (owing to their oily nature), being as injurious as salmon. In respect to vegetables, not only should potatoes be prohibited, but parsnips, beetroot, turnips, and carrots. The truth is, I seldom or ever partook of these objectionable articles myself, and did not reflect that others might do so, or that they were forbidden. Green vegetables are considered very beneficial, and I believe should be adopted at all times. I am indebted to the "Cornhill Magazine" and other journals for drawing my attention to these dietetic points. I can now also state that eggs, if not hard boiled, are unexceptionable, that cheese, if sparingly used, and plain boiled rice seem harmless.

Some doubts have been expressed in regard to the vanishing point of such a descending scale, but it is a remarkable fact that the great and most palpable diminution in weight and bulk occurs within the first forty-eight hours, the descent is then more gradual. My own experience, and that of others, assures me (if medical authority be first consulted as to the complaint) that with such slight extraneous aid as medicine can afford, nature will do her duty, and only her duty: firstly, by relieving herself of immediate pressure she will be enabled to move more freely in her own beautiful way, and secondly, by pursuing the same course to work speedy amelioration and final cure. The vanishing point is only when the disease is stopped and the parasite annihilated.

It may interest my readers to know that I have now apparently attained the standard natural at my age (10 stone 10, or 150 lbs.), as my weight now varies only to the extent of 1lb., more or less, in the course of a month. According to Dr. Hutchinson's tables I ought to lose still more, but cannot do so without resorting to medicine; and, feeling in sound vigorous health, I am perfectly content to wait upon nature for any further change.

In my humble judgment the dietary is the principal point in the treatment of Corpulence, and it appears to me, moreover, that if properly regulated it becomes in a certain sense a medicine. The system seems to me to attack only the superfluous deposit of fat, and, as my medical friend informs me, purges the blood, rendering it more pure and healthy, strengthens the muscles and bodily viscera, and I feel quite convinced sweetens life, if it does not prolong it.

It is truly gratifying to me to be able now to add that many other of the most exalted members of the Faculty have honoured my movement in the question with their approbation.

I consider it a public duty further to state, that Mr. Harvey, whom I have named in the 43rd page as my kind medical adviser in the cure of Corpulence, is not Dr. John Harvey, who has published a Pamphlet on Corpulence assimilating with some of the features and the general aspect of mine, and which has been considered (as I learn from correspondents who have obtained it) the work of my medical friend. It is not.

I am glad, therefore, to repeat that my medical adviser was, and is still, Mr WILLIAM HARVEY, F.R.C.S., No. 2, Soho Square, London, W.

WILLIAM BANTING

April, 1864.

WILLIAM BANTING

PREFACE TO THE FOURTH EDITION

Some five years after producing the Third Edition of
Letter on Corpulence, Banting issued a Fourth Edition.
This 1869 edition was to be the last to be printed in his
lifetime. He was to die 9 years later at his home in
Kensington having lived until the remarkable age of 81.
The preface (abridged) to this Fourth Edition is included
here as it offers some interesting insight into the resistance
and criticism that Banting met following publication of the
earlier editions. His method was attacked, his medical
knowledge questioned (he never claimed to have any!) and
perhaps most upsetting to Banting himself – his motives
for producing his letter were speculated upon. In this
preface, Banting lays bare his financial accounts for the
project. He details the costs, the income and the profit
made and – to finally silence his critics - he details the
good causes that benefited from the distribution of those
very same profits. With obvious glee he declares "so
much...for the fortune...I have made!"

WILLIAM BANTING

FOURTH EDITION

WITH PREFATORY REMARKS BY THE AUTHOR

COPIOUS INFORMATION FROM CORRESPONDENTS AND CONFIRMATORY EVIDENCE OF THE

BENEFIT OF THE DIETARY SYSTEM WHICH HE RECOMMENDED TO PUBLIC NOTICE

WILLIAM BANTING

It is with no slight degree of pride and satisfaction that I presume to publish a fourth edition of my Letter on Corpulence, in the hope and belief that it may still further interest and benefit the Public. The preceding editions were composed and issued with all sorts of apparent defects and deformities from my utter inability to afford any *substantial* evidence of the merit and utility of the system beyond my own personal and short experience. Five years have now elapsed since the third edition was published. It has happily attained a world-wide circulation, and afforded me a vast amount of pleasure and gratification, derived from the conviction that I have been the means of bringing under public consideration and discussion one of the little known and much neglected laws of nature. The popularity of my unpretending *brochure* is manifest, not only in the surprising sale of no less than 63,000 copies, in this country alone, but by its translation into foreign languages and its large and rapid circulation in France, Germany, and the United States. In addition to this I have received nearly 2,000 very complimentary and grateful letters from all quarters of the world.

Feeling intense interest in a thorough examination of this important question, I solicited correspondence, in order that I might obtain the fullest information from the experience of others. This, of course, has consumed a great deal of my time, as well as occasioned considerable expense. Fortunately, however, I had leisure, inclination, and means at my disposal, and considered it a privilege to employ them in the service of my fellow-creatures. The correspondence has been a great source of interest to myself, and I believe will likewise interest and benefit the public at large.

The great principle which Mr. William Harvey (my medical adviser), of Soho Square, inculcated, having been confirmed by my own personal experience, I was enabled to speak with perfect confidence, and I became invulnerable to the ridicule, contempt, or abuse which were not spared in the earlier stages of the discussion. I believe I have subdued my discourteous assailants by silence and patience; and I can now look with pity, not unmixed with sorrow, upon men of eminence who had the rashness and folly to designate the dietary system as "humbug," and to hold up to scorn the man who put it forth, although he never derived nor sought pecuniary or personal recompense, but simply desired, out of gratitude, to make known to other sufferers the remedy which he had found so efficacious to himself. I heartily thank the public press for the general fairness of its criticisms, and feel deeply indebted to the *Morning Advertiser* for its able article on 3rd October, 1865, when I was so sadly and unjustly attacked by certain prominent members of the British Association, whose feelings, now that the subject has been more widely and intelligently discussed, I do not envy.

My sole objects in issuing a fourth edition are -

First.- *To* offer my further personal experience on the subject since I published the third edition in 1864.

Secondly.--To adduce some remarkable proofs of the benefits afforded to others by the dietary system, in verification of my own testimony.

Thirdly.-To apply any profits which may arise from its sale to various charitable objects, after the plan I followed with the unexpected gains of the third edition.

I have been strongly and frequently advised to publish some of the highly interesting reports I have received from correspondents, in proof of the great value of a proper dietary system in advanced life, and of the soundness of Mr. William Harvey's advice, which proved so beneficial to me; but I have hitherto refrained from doing so, under the belief that if the statement of my own personal experience was not credited, no weight would be attached to any other evidence which I could adduce. At length, however, I have yielded to the suggestion, and can only hope that this accumulated and unimpeachable evidence may prove interesting and convincing, even to the most resolute unbeliever.

It has been reported to me that many medical men have argued that I could not have consulted any eminent members of their fraternity on the subject of obesity. I beg leave emphatically to assure the public that, for the 20 years, previous to consulting Mr. Harvey, I had no occasion to consult a medical man, for any other ailments except those which are the inevitable consequences of corpulence; and that, although my medical advisers were neither few, nor of second-rate reputation, not one of them pointed out the real cause of my sufferings, nor proposed any effectual remedy, until I appealed to my friend, Mr. Harvey, the celebrated aurist, on account *only* of deafness.

I will not affirm that I said to each "pray remove my corpulence," for I had been told that it was, and really thought it to be, incurable; but all my disorders resulted from it, and Mr. Harvey was the first to acquaint me with the fact.

It is possible, and I think probable, that even Mr. Harvey was somewhat surprised at the extraordinary and speedy result of my rigid adherence to his advice, because he had long before prescribed the proper dietary system to reduce or cure corpulence, but his patients having hitherto imprudently slighted his prescriptions, it was only my very strict compliance that completely proved the accuracy of his judgment. My only merit consists in entire obedience to Mr. Harvey's advice. To him alone belongs all the credit of the remedy. He was the first to lead me on to the true road of health, and I was probably the first of his many patients who kept to it.

I have never assumed the slightest medical knowledge, but, on the contrary, I have assured every correspondent that I was utterly ignorant of the physiological or chemical reasons for the wonderful results produced by the prescribed dietary; nor do I come before the public now with any pretensions whatever to such knowledge, but simply to offer my five past years' experience in confirmation of my original observations upon the great fact, backed by the experience of numerous correspondents in all classes of society, male and female, in the hope that the evidence which I have collected may induce medical and scientific men to promote a still wider knowledge of this important truth, *"that change of diet is frequently necessary in advancing and advanced Isle to secure good bodily health and comfort, particularly to the corpulent and obese."*

It was unfortunate, and doubtless detrimental, in the early stages of my crusade against Corpulence, that theoretical writers in *Blackwood's Edinburgh Magazine,* and other influential periodicals, should have dwelt so strongly upon my four meals a day, *presuming they were four heavy meals.* No part of my pamphlet states this. Since attaining manhood I have been rather remarkable for the moderation of my meals, and I very much doubt if any man, in sound health., and actively occupied, has consumed less in the course of the twenty-four hours. I am thoroughly convinced, that it is QUALITY alone which requires notice, and not *quantity.* This has been emphatically denied by some writers in the public papers, but I can confidently assert, upon the indisputable evidence of many of my correspondents, as well as my own, that they are mistaken. I apprehend that people of larger frame and build may require a proportionately larger quantity of the prescribed diet, but they must be guided by their own judgment in the application of the principles laid down.

It was probably my misfortune, never to have heard of a celebrated work, *La Physiologie du Goût,* by Brillat Savarin, and other treatises by Bernard and Dancel; but I had full confidence that our own eminent medical men (second to none in Europe) were well informed of every new scientific fact discovered in Paris or elsewhere, and I never dreamed of consulting those foreign authorities, from whom, as the public press has since informed me, I might have obtained a remedy for the cure of Corpulence.

My unpretending letter on Corpulence has at least brought all these facts to the surface for public examination, and they have thereby had already a great share of attention, and will doubtless receive much more until the system is thoroughly understood and properly appreciated by every thinking man and woman in the civilized world.

I have been told, again and again, that the system was as old as the hills. I will not deny it, because I cannot; but I can say for myself and my many correspondents, that it was q*uite new to us;* or some of us would doubtless have been recommended to practise it by medical advisers, as I have no doubt they are now, and as they surely will be hereafter more extensively.

Some writers have assumed that I had no great grievance in my corpulent state. Are failing sight and hearing, an umbilical rupture requiring a truss, bandages for weak knees and ankles, not serious grievances? Those only who have suffered from corpulence can adequately understand its miseries or appreciate the merits of a system so admirably adapted to its relief.

My earnest, and indeed my only desire throughout has been to ventilate this question in the interest of humanity, and to ascertain not only the advantages of the system now called "Banting," but also any possible mischief in its application, and I am bound to say, that I have not met *with any case where* harm *has ensued from its practice under medical authority and supervision.* Two or three unfavourable results having been reported in the public papers, I instantly set to work to trace them, and proved them to have no better foundation than the frequent reports of my *death.* I may admit that about a month after the issue of the third edition, I received an abusive letter on the subject from an anonymous correspondent, who may flatter himself that he has preserved his incognito, but I venture to assure him that *he has not,* and that his abuse is no argument against the system, but simply a proof of his own want of manners and common sense.

In my desire to get at the whole truth, I sent a copy of my pamphlet to some of the leading professional men of the day, and I have received several kind and practical replies. A few of these will be found among the evidences I offer. One of these testimonies I cannot resist quoting here as well:

"The rules of diet you found so beneficial have long been "forced upon men who are under training for running, or "prize fights; apparently, however, their especial efficacy "was overlooked, because other rules relating to exercise, "sweating, &c., were mixed up with them."

This plain, simple statement, in my opinion, unlocks the whole mystery, and solves the problem which had long slumbered, until my perseverance under Mr. Harvey's treatment happily brought it under complete examination.

No doubt the system was known, and had been practised, but only to promote muscular vigour in healthy people, for special objects, yet had never been applied to the unhealthy and corpulent, because it was impossible for such people to take the necessary exercise and sweating. It is now proved that, by *proper diet alone,* the evils of corpulence may be removed without the addition of those active exercises, which are impossible to the sickly or unwieldy patient.

Another eminent medical man, whose letter will appear among the rest, was actually giving my pamphlets in the course of his practice. I was greatly surprised to hear of it, and wrote to ascertain the fact. He invited me to call on him, and showed me that my information was correct by pointing to a pile of them lying upon his table. He complimented me upon the publication, as it contained sound advice in cases like my own; and added, that the discovery was not Mr. Harvey's, but was derived from "Mons. Bernard, of Paris." I replied that Mr. Harvey had told me he had first derived his information from lectures which he had heard in Paris, by Mons. Bernard, in regard to diabetes, and some other complaints, but that he had himself applied it to cases of corpulency. He admitted that the simple record of my own experience of the value of the system had brought it to the clear light of day, and that if it had been written by a medical man, it would scarcely have been noticed by the general public at all.

Probably no one was ever subjected to more ridicule and abuse than I have been, in English as well as in foreign journals. My only object, however, has been the good of my fellow creatures. To have accomplished this object, in any degree, is a sufficient reward for my expenditure of time and means, and an ample compensation for the insolent contempt of some, and the feeble ribaldry of others.

I certainly was somewhat astonished at one time, and not a little amused, to find that my death was generally reported, even to myself~ by some who did not happen to know me personally; and, at another, to hear that I had been seriously ill and afflicted with boils, carbuncles, and other ailments, through my rigid pursuit of the dietary system. 1 am, therefore, glad of this opportunity to state publicly (what hundreds of my friends can attest) that I do not know what gout or a headache is, that I have always ate, drank, and slept well, have had no carbuncles, boils, or any real illness whatever, since I began the system recommended by Mr. Harvey; indeed, the only ailment which I have had, was a little additional eruption in my hands in 1867, a discomfort by which I had been more or less troubled for years, but from which I was soon relieved, doubtless, by the continued pursuit of the dietary system. I have, therefore, offered no nostrum or quack remedy, but have simply stated the results of my following professional advice, and have only claimed for it a thorough examination by the public, and our highly intelligent medical professors; indeed, I recommended all *to consult their medical advisers* be fore adopting what I individually considered a perfectly harmless system. I knew nothing of causes, physiological or chemical, for the wondrous effects produced by a generous, in exchange for a meagre, dietary; but believed, as I still believe, that it is a simple remedy to reduce and destroy superfluous fat; that it may be an alleviation, if not a cure, of gout; that it prevents or eradicates carbuncles, boils, and the elements of dyspepsia; makes advanced life more enjoyable, and promotes longevity. I consider my general health extraordinary; indeed, I meet with few men at 72 years of age who have so little cause to complain. I trust, therefore, that if any future adverse reports of my health and condition should arise, they may be communicated to me through the Post-office, that I may be able at once to contradict, if possible, such silly rumours. I cannot, now, retract anything I have written on the subject, and hence the publication of a fourth edition, *condensed,* with such observations as five years' subsequent experience enables me to offer in verification of its general honesty and truth.

I have no doubt there is already a considerable reduction in the number of my corpulent and otherwise afflicted brethren, through the rigid or even partial adherence to the dietary called "Banting," but I have seen still *far* too many in my rambles about England, and to all such I trust the publication of a fourth edition of my pamphlet may be useful. I earnestly recommend any so afflicted, who choose to make trial of the system, to be accurately weighed, after consulting some medical adviser, before beginning it; and, again, at the end of seven days, during which short period the chief and most extraordinary diminution of weight occurs. This will be ample time to convince the most sceptical of its merit and utility, an(I thereby give increased confidence to its further pursuit, under medical sanction. So short a trial of superior in exchange for inferior, or more simple diet, can surely do no great harm to the human frame, should the grievance arise from other causes than undue corpulence; but I believe medical men will be found in all quarters of the world who have been induced to investigate this important subject of late years, and that in consequence the public generally will now be more properly advised on the subject.

It is, perhaps, of small consequence to the public, but it is a question of great importance to me, to show that I have kept faith with them, and may be relied upon for the future I therefore invite their attention to the cost of the publication, and to the manner in which the profits have been expended.

The first edition of 1,000 copies of my pamphlet I presented to clubs, learned and medical societies, and to the public. The second edition, or 1,000 copies, I also gave to the public; and 500 copies of the last I directed to be sold for the benefit of my Printers' Sick Fund, as I found that some preferred to purchase them.

These, and the distribution, cost me about £40, for which I did not expect or receive one penny in return.

I was advised that, to pay for the expense of printing, publishing, and advertising a third edition, of 20,000 copies, I should charge for them one shilling each, but as pecuniary advantage was neither my desire nor aim, I determined to issue them at sixpence each, and rather lose by it than think of profit. The sale, however, increased so wonderfully, that at the end of eight months 50,000 copies were sold, with a result which the press kindly published at the time.

Since that period 13,000 more copies have been sold, and I have increased pleasure and satisfaction in reporting the following total result

	£ s.d.	
Received- By the sale of 63,000	58,154	or
copies, as 4,846 dozens, and 2 copies,		
according to the trade custom, at 4s.		
per dozen	969 4 8	

Paid- £ s.d.
For setting, correcting, casting,
and printing 63,000 copies,
bound in wrappers .. 633 13 0

	£ s.d.	£ s.d.
Brought forward ..	633 13 0	969 4 8
For advertising in the London		
and country papers, and		
incidental expenses ..	110 1 8	743 14 8

Leaving a profit to the Author of .. £225 10 0

which I have had the gratification of distributing as follows

	£ s.d.
To The Printers' Pension Society, at the	
Anniversary Dinner, in March, 1864,	
per Chas. Dickens, Esq.	50 0 0
Ditto, subsequently	21 0 0

The Royal Hospital for Incurables..	50 0 0
The British Home for Incurables..	50 0 0
The National Orthopœdic Hospital..	10 10 0
The City of London Truss Society..	10 10 0
The West London Hospital	10 10 0
The Great Northern Hospital	10 10 0
The Epileptic Hospital	10 10 0
The Alexandra Institution for the Blind	10 10 0
The Sick Fund of Morning Advertiser	5 0 0
The Sick Fund of my Printers' Estab'	5 0 0

£225 10 0

So much as regards the fortune which it was very generally reported that I had made by the "speculation"!!

It may possibly interest the public to know the result of my own proceedings and personal experience since I published my third edition in 1864. My weight has continued at about 11 stone, from which I have never varied more or less than 3 lbs., principally when I was experimenting to ascertain my own greatest dietetic enemy; and I have proved very satisfactorily that it is and was sugar and saccharine elements.

I have ascertained, by repeated experiments, that five ounces of sugar distributed equally over seven days, which is not an ounce per (lay, will augment my weight nearly one pound by the end of that short period. The other forbidden elements have not produced so extraordinary a result. In these, therefore, I am not so rigid. Some people (as will be seen by their letters) find other things detrimental. I never eat bread unless it is stale, cut thin, and well. toasted. I very seldom take any butter, certainly not a pound in a year. I seldom take milk (though that called so, in London, is probably misnamed), and I am quite sure that I do not drink a gallon of it in the whole year. I occasionally eat a potato with my dinner, possibly to the extent of 1 lb. per week. I spoke of sherry as very admissible, and I am glad of this opportunity to say, that I have since discovered it promoted acidity. Perhaps the best sherry I could procure was not the *very* best, but I found weak light claret, or brandy, gin, and whisky, with water, suited me better; and I have been led to believe that fruit, however ripe, does not suit me so well taken raw as when cooked, without sugar. I find that vegetables of all kinds, grown above ground, ripened to maturity and well boiled, are admirable; but I avoid all roots, as carrot, turnip, parsnip, and beet. I have not taken any kind of medicine for eighteen months, and find that my dietary contains all the needful regimen which my system requires. In the firm belief and conviction that the *quality* in food is the chief desideratum, and that the question of *quantity* is mere moonshine, I take the most agreeable and savoury viands, meat and game pies, that my cook can concoct, with the best possible gravies, jellies, &c., the fat being skimmed off; but I never, or very rarely, take a morsel of pie or pudding crusts.

My bodily organization *may* be somewhat different from that of others; but the facts which I have related are indisputable, for they are the result of my own personal experience, which I have made known for the benefit of others who have suffered, as I have done, and whose testimony of the efficacy of the remedy confirms my own.

Being fond of green peas, I take them daily in the season, and I gain 2 or 3 lbs. in weight as well as some little in bulk, but I soon lose both when their season is over. For this trespass I quite forgive myself.

The subjoined correspondence is only a portion of upwards of 1,800 letters which I have received. There is scarcely one out of the whole which does not breathe a spirit of pure thankfulness and gratitude for the benefits derived from the dietary system, and contain the most flattering encomiums on my character and motives. One or two, indeed, of a totally opposite character have reached me, and I would not have refrained from publishing them, had the writers not thought proper to deprive them of any authority by concealing their names. I had originally selected a much larger number for publication, but I fear that even these few may be tiresome to some readers, though I have abridged them as far as possible by omitting personal compliments, and irrelevant matter and enquiries, &c., of little importance to any but the writers. They will, however, I believe, be perused with interest by many others, who can select such facts from them as may apply to their own special cases.

A great many of these correspondents—indeed, some of the most interesting—have granted me full permission to print their names and addresses, in verification, and I have no doubt whatever that I could obtain the consent of nearly all to the free publication of their letters; but I consider it quite unnecessary to give more than the number and date of the respective letters, assuring the reader that these extracts have been faithfully made, and that I am ready to produce the originals to any person who applies to inc in good faith and honesty of purpose to examine still further this very important subject.

I could certainly have wished that the crowning proof of the veracity and utility of my statements had emanated from one of my own countrymen, but it was not to be, although one of them, as I have shown, unlocked the mystery and so far solved the great problem. I am indebted to a foreigner for this efficient service; and I now, in conclusion, request particular attention to the last article in this pamphlet, namely,—a lecture given before the King and Court of Wurtemburg, at Stuttgart, in December 1865, by the celebrated physician and professor, Dr. Niemeyer, which I have had very carefully translated.

I heartily thank that generous and able man for the valuable testimony which he has borne to the truth of the system, for the honour and credit which he has bestowed upon my medical adviser, Mr. William Harvey, and for his gratifying tribute to my own motives and conduct in publishing my experience to the world.

WILLIAM BANTING.

Kensington,
May, 1869.

ABOUT THE AUTHORS

William Banting

William Banting (c. December 1796-16 March 1878) was a well known London Funeral Director. His family business served the Royal Household for much of the 19th Century and Banting conducted the funerals of King George III, King George IV, the Duke of Wellington and Prince Albert. The family business would continue after his death and go on to arrange the funerals of Prince Leopold and Queen Victoria.

Despite his success as a Funeral Director, Banting is most well known for his 1863 book *Letter on Corpulence*. The book detailed Banting's struggle with obesity, the impact this had on his health and – importantly – the measures he took to lose weight and regain his health.

Letter on Corpulence became a huge success, was published internationally, and ran into five editions in the UK - the last being published posthumously in 1902.

WILLIAM BANTING

Will Meadows

Will Meadows was born and grew up in a once-proud South Yorkshire town. Much of his working life has been spent travelling the globe and he has a particular fondness for Asia.

His career has spanned a number of industries with the majority of his experience in the fields of diet and nutrition.

Will has authored a number of magazine and journal articles. A distillation of Will's personal and working experiences can be found in his own diet book *The Final Countdown Diet*.

Will lives in West Yorkshire in a village closely linked with food. He lives with his wife Jane and their three children. Will speaks, and eats, Chinese.

WILLIAM BANTING

ALSO BY WILL MEADOWS

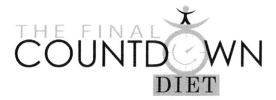

"The last diet book you will ever need to buy"

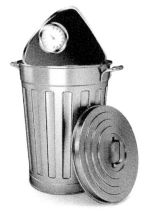

**AN INSIDER'S GUIDE TO WHY DIETS FAIL
& THE SECRETS OF
PERMANENT FAT LOSS**

Will Meadows

www.finalcountdowndiet.com

Notes

Notes

Notes

Notes

Notes

Notes

Notes

Printed in Great Britain
by Amazon